The Lady Era Handbook

A Journey through Women's Health and the Evolution of Hormonal Treatments and Exploring the Impact of Hormone Therapy on Women's Lives and Wellness across Generations.

Shirley McIntosh

© Copyright 2024 Shirley McIntosh.

All rights reserved.

Disclaimer

The information provided in this book is for educsational purposes only and is not intended as medical advice. The content is based on current research and best practices at the time of publication. However, it may not reflect the most recent developments in medicine or individual patient circumstances.

Readers are strongly encouraged to consult with a qualified healthcare professional before making any changes to their medical regimen or treatment plans. The authors and publishers of this book are not liable for any adverse effects or consequences resulting from the use or misuse of the information contained herein.

Always seek the advice of your physician or other qualified health provider with any questions you may have regarding a medical condition or treatment. If you are experiencing a medical emergency, call emergency services immediately.

Table of Contents

Introduction 1

Chapter One 4
Historical Context 4

Chapter Two 9
The Science behind Lady Era Drugs 9

Chapter Three 15
Types of Lady Era Drugs 15

Chapter Four 21
Safety and Side Effects 21

Chapter Five 26
Societal Implications 26

Chapter Six 31
Personal Experiences: Societal Implications 31

Introduction

In recent years, discussions surrounding women's sexual health have gained significant attention, revealing a complex landscape that has often been overshadowed by historical stigma and misunderstanding. The quest for sexual wellness is not merely a personal journey; it reflects broader societal attitudes toward female desire, autonomy, and health. Among the various approaches to enhancing sexual well-being, the emergence of Lady Era drugs has sparked a wave of curiosity and controversy, raising important questions about their role in women's lives.

Historically, the conversation around female sexuality has been fraught with challenges. For centuries, women's sexual needs and desires were often dismissed or pathologized, categorized as taboo or inappropriate. This narrative persisted through the ages, from the Victorian era's strict moral codes to the more modern stigmatization of women seeking pleasure or expressing their sexual desires. As a result, many women have found themselves navigating a landscape that is, at times, hostile to their needs, leaving them feeling isolated and misunderstood.

With the advent of Lady Era drugs—medications designed specifically to address issues like hypoactive sexual desire disorder (HSDD)—the landscape is beginning to shift. These drugs represent a breakthrough in medical research and a growing acknowledgment of women's sexual health as a legitimate area of study. As scientists and healthcare professionals work to develop and refine these medications, they aim to provide women with the tools to reclaim their sexual health and well-being, fundamentally altering the narrative surrounding female desire.

However, the introduction of these drugs is not without controversy. While many women celebrate the availability of options that address their sexual health concerns, others express caution. The discourse often centers around the effectiveness of these medications, the potential side effects, and the ethical implications of pharmaceutical interventions in intimate aspects of life. Moreover, the commercialization of female sexual health raises questions about the commodification of desire and the potential for exploitation in a market eager to meet the demand for enhancement.

The societal implications are profound. The conversation about Lady Era drugs is not just about individual health; it reflects deeper issues of gender equity in healthcare, the role of women in society, and the ongoing battle against the stigmatization of female sexuality. For too long, women's sexual health has been marginalized within the broader healthcare system, often overshadowed by the emphasis on male sexual health. This imbalance has fueled a cultural narrative that devalues women's experiences, perpetuating a cycle of silence and shame.

As we delve deeper into the complexities of Lady Era drugs, it is essential to recognize the diverse experiences of women who seek them. Each woman's journey is unique, shaped by her own cultural, social, and personal context. The decision to pursue medication for sexual enhancement can be empowering, allowing women to take control of their bodies and their sexual health. Yet, it can also be fraught with anxiety and uncertainty, as women grapple with societal expectations, personal desires, and medical advice.

In this book, we will explore the multifaceted nature of Lady Era drugs, examining their historical context, scientific foundations, and personal narratives. We aim to provide a comprehensive understanding that transcends mere pharmacology, engaging with the emotional, psychological, and societal dimensions of women's sexual health. By doing so, we hope to foster a more nuanced conversation about female desire, empowering women to make informed choices about their bodies and their sexual well-being.

The journey toward understanding Lady Era drugs is also a journey toward reclaiming the narrative around women's sexuality—transforming it from one of shame and silence into one of empowerment and open dialogue. As we navigate through the complexities of this topic, we invite readers to join us in exploring the intersections of medicine, society, and personal experience, ultimately fostering a more inclusive and supportive environment for women everywhere.

Chapter One

Historical Context

The historical context of women's sexual health is a tapestry woven from threads of culture, science, and societal norms, reflecting a complex evolution that has shaped contemporary attitudes and medical practices. Understanding this history is crucial for grasping the significance of Lady Era drugs and the discourse surrounding female sexuality today.

From ancient civilizations to modern times, the perception of female sexuality has oscillated between reverence and repression. In many early societies, women were often seen as embodiments of fertility and life, celebrated for their reproductive capabilities. Cultures such as those in ancient Egypt and Greece recognized the power of female sexuality, associating it with goddess figures who symbolized both pleasure and fertility. Yet, even within these cultures, the narrative around women's sexual autonomy was constrained by patriarchal structures that defined acceptable behavior and desires.

As societies evolved, particularly during the Middle Ages, the attitude towards female sexuality took a marked turn. With the rise of Christianity, a more restrictive view emerged, characterizing women's sexual desires as sinful or inherently flawed. This era instilled a sense of shame around female sexuality, promoting ideals of chastity and purity. Women were often vilified for expressing sexual desires, leading to a cultural climate where discussions of female pleasure became taboo. The societal implications of this shift were profound, as women's sexual health was largely ignored within the medical community, relegated to whispers and secrecy.

The Enlightenment and the subsequent Victorian era brought about a new wave of thought, yet many of the underlying attitudes towards female sexuality remained entrenched. Although the period witnessed advancements in science and philosophy, women's sexual health was often framed in the context of morality rather than biology. Medical professionals frequently pathologized female sexual desire, labeling it as hysteria or neurosis, a condition that required treatment rather than understanding. This misguided approach not only misrepresented women's experiences but also solidified a narrative that women should suppress their desires.

As the 20th century dawned, the landscape began to shift with the emergence of feminist movements advocating for women's rights and sexual liberation. Pioneering figures such as Margaret Sanger campaigned for birth control and reproductive rights, emphasizing the importance of women's autonomy over their bodies. This era of activism laid the groundwork for future discussions about female sexuality, encouraging women to assert their rights and challenge societal norms. However, even as these movements gained traction, the medical community remained slow to adapt. Many physicians continued to overlook the distinct sexual health needs of women, focusing instead on male-centric perspectives.

The sexual revolution of the 1960s and 1970s marked a significant turning point in the conversation around women's sexuality. As cultural norms shifted, women began to reclaim their sexual agency, advocating for both pleasure and health. This period saw the rise of comprehensive sex education and the introduction of contraceptive methods, empowering women to take control of their reproductive choices. However, despite these advances, medical research on female sexuality lagged behind. While erectile dysfunction medications were developed for men, women were largely left without comparable options for addressing their sexual health concerns.

In the late 20th century, researchers and activists began to call attention to the neglect of women's sexual health within medical discourse. The recognition of hypoactive sexual desire disorder (HSDD) emerged as a critical focal point, highlighting the need for treatments that addressed women's sexual health issues. This period marked the beginning of a more concerted effort to study female sexual function and desire, paving the way for the development of Lady Era drugs.

The introduction of flibanserin in the early 2010s as a treatment for HSDD was a watershed moment. For the first time, women had a pharmacological option specifically designed to enhance sexual desire, a stark contrast to the plethora of treatments available for men. The approval of this drug sparked both celebration and controversy, igniting debates about the medicalization of female sexuality and the implications of introducing pharmaceutical interventions into an intimate aspect of life. Proponents argued that it was a significant step towards acknowledging women's sexual health needs, while critics voiced concerns about the potential side effects, efficacy, and the broader implications of normalizing drug use for sexual enhancement.

The discussions surrounding Lady Era drugs are now intertwined with ongoing conversations about gender equity in healthcare. The historical neglect of women's sexual health has resulted in a landscape where women's voices are often sidelined, even as they seek treatment and understanding. As we explore the development and impact of Lady Era drugs, it is vital to consider not only the medical and scientific aspects but also the social and cultural narratives that continue to influence perceptions of female desire.

As we progress through this narrative, it is important to remember that the journey toward understanding women's sexual health is ongoing. The history of Lady Era drugs is not just about the science of medication; it is also about the empowerment of women to take control of their sexual health and advocate for their needs. The evolution of this discourse reflects broader societal changes, revealing the power dynamics at play and the necessity of dismantling barriers that have historically limited women's access to comprehensive sexual health care.

This chapter serves as a foundation for understanding the context in which Lady Era drugs have emerged, shedding light on the cultural attitudes that have shaped women's experiences and health needs throughout history. It is a journey marked by struggle, resilience, and a gradual awakening to the importance of women's sexual health—an awakening that continues to evolve as society becomes more attuned to the complexities of female desire. In the following chapters, we will explore the scientific underpinnings of these medications, their societal implications, and the personal narratives of women who navigate the intersection of health, desire, and empowerment in the modern world.

Chapter Two

The Science behind Lady Era Drugs

Understanding the science behind Lady Era drugs involves delving into the intricate interplay of biology, psychology, and pharmacology. These medications, designed primarily to address hypoactive sexual desire disorder (HSDD) and related issues, represent a significant step in the evolution of treatments aimed at enhancing female sexual health. To grasp their efficacy and implications, one must first explore the underlying biological mechanisms of female sexuality, the specific medications developed, and the ongoing research efforts aimed at refining these treatments.

At the core of female sexual desire lies a complex web of hormonal, neurological, and psychological factors. Unlike male sexual function, which is often more straightforward due to the hormonal surge associated with testosterone, female sexuality is influenced by a multitude of factors that can fluctuate over time. Hormones like estrogen and progesterone play significant roles, affecting libido in various phases of a woman's life—from menstruation and pregnancy to menopause. This hormonal interplay is further complicated by neurotransmitters in the brain, such as dopamine and serotonin, which can enhance or inhibit sexual desire and arousal.

Research has shown that dopamine, often termed the "pleasure neurotransmitter," is closely linked to motivation and reward. In contrast, serotonin is associated with mood regulation and can sometimes dampen sexual desire. The balance between these neurotransmitters is crucial; for instance, low levels of dopamine or elevated levels of serotonin can lead to diminished libido. Understanding these biochemical pathways is essential for developing effective treatments for sexual dysfunction, as medications must target specific mechanisms to restore balance and enhance sexual desire.

The introduction of Lady Era drugs, particularly flibanserin and bremelanotide, has been groundbreaking in this context. Flibanserin, initially developed as an antidepressant, was later found to have effects on sexual desire. It acts primarily on the brain's neurotransmitter systems by increasing dopamine levels while simultaneously decreasing serotonin levels. This dual action is designed to enhance sexual desire in premenopausal women diagnosed with HSDD.

Clinical trials evaluating flibanserin's effectiveness revealed that it could lead to an increase in the number of satisfying sexual events and an overall improvement in sexual desire. However, the path to its approval was not without controversy. Critics questioned the modest benefits compared to the side effects, which included dizziness, fatigue, and nausea. The FDA's eventual approval in

2015 was a watershed moment, yet it underscored the broader debate about medicalizing female sexual desire.

Bremelanotide, another drug approved for HSDD, takes a different approach. It is a peptide that acts on melanocortin receptors in the brain, stimulating pathways associated with sexual arousal and desire. Bremelanotide is administered via subcutaneous injection, and its approval in 2019 offered women a new option that directly targets the neurobiology of sexual function. Unlike flibanserin, which needs to be taken daily, bremelanotide is used on an as-needed basis, providing flexibility for women seeking to enhance their sexual experiences.

The introduction of these drugs marks a significant milestone in the understanding of female sexual health, yet the science is still evolving. Ongoing research seeks to uncover further nuances in female desire and arousal, exploring how various factors, including psychological aspects and life experiences, interact with biological mechanisms. For example, studies are increasingly recognizing the role of contextual factors—such as relationship dynamics, stress, and mental health—in shaping a woman's sexual desire.

A crucial aspect of this ongoing research involves understanding individual variability. Not every woman responds the same way to these medications, which can lead to questions about personalized medicine in the realm of sexual health. Factors such as genetics, lifestyle, and underlying health conditions can all influence how a woman experiences sexual desire and how she responds to treatment. Researchers are now looking into pharmacogenomics—the study of how genes affect a person's response to drugs—to better tailor treatments to individual needs.

Moreover, the focus is expanding beyond just pharmacological solutions. Researchers are increasingly investigating the impact of non-pharmaceutical interventions, such as cognitive-behavioral therapy (CBT) and couples therapy, in addressing issues related to sexual desire. These therapies can provide women with tools to navigate the emotional and relational complexities that often accompany sexual dysfunction. By combining pharmacological treatments with psychological support, healthcare providers can offer a more holistic approach to enhancing female sexual health.

The scientific exploration of Lady Era drugs also raises important ethical questions. As society grapples with the medicalization of female sexuality, discussions are increasingly focused on the implications of using drugs to enhance desire. Critics argue that pharmaceuticals should not be the primary solution for addressing what may be complex emotional or relational issues. The concern is that this focus on medication could overshadow the importance of comprehensive sexual health education, open communication about sexual needs, and the exploration of non-drug interventions.

Another area of concern is the potential for societal pressures to dictate the need for these medications. As women navigate societal expectations around sexuality and pleasure, the availability of drugs designed to enhance desire could lead to unrealistic standards of sexual performance and satisfaction. The risk lies in creating an environment where women feel compelled to seek pharmacological solutions to fit into prescribed ideals of femininity and sexuality.

As we continue to examine the science behind Lady Era drugs, it is essential to maintain an open dialogue about these issues. Women should be empowered to make informed choices about their sexual health, understanding the benefits and limitations of available treatments. The goal should be to foster an environment where women can openly discuss their desires and experiences without stigma, encouraging a more nuanced understanding of what sexual health means.

In conclusion, the science behind Lady Era drugs reflects a convergence of biological, psychological, and social dimensions that influence female sexual health. As research continues to evolve, it is crucial to consider the implications of these medications not only as treatments for sexual dysfunction but also as part of a broader discourse on women's rights, health, and autonomy. By fostering a comprehensive understanding of female sexuality, we can help ensure that women receive the care and support they need to thrive—both in their sexual health and their overall well-being. In the subsequent chapters, we will explore the societal implications of these drugs, personal narratives, and alternative approaches that empower women to take control of their sexual health journeys.

Chapter Three

Types of Lady Era Drugs

The landscape of Lady Era drugs is both diverse and complex, reflecting the multifaceted nature of female sexuality and the various factors that can influence a woman's sexual health. This chapter will explore the prominent types of medications designed to address issues such as hypoactive sexual desire disorder (HSDD) and other related conditions. Each drug not only represents a unique approach to enhancing female sexual desire but also encapsulates the broader journey of understanding and addressing women's health needs.

At the forefront of this discussion is flibanserin, the first medication specifically approved to treat HSDD in premenopausal women. Initially developed as an antidepressant, flibanserin operates through a multifaceted mechanism of action, primarily targeting neurotransmitter systems in the brain. It acts as a serotonin 1A receptor agonist and a serotonin 2A receptor antagonist, which helps balance the neurotransmitter levels that influence sexual desire. By increasing dopamine and norepinephrine levels while reducing serotonin, flibanserin aims to enhance a woman's sexual appetite.

Flibanserin's clinical trials were significant in demonstrating its efficacy, with studies revealing an increase in the number of satisfying sexual experiences among women who took the medication. However, the journey to its approval was contentious. Critics raised concerns about its side effects, including dizziness, fatigue, and potential interactions with alcohol. These concerns were compounded by debates about the appropriateness of pharmaceutical intervention for what some viewed as a complex interplay of psychological, relational, and biological factors. Nevertheless, flibanserin's approval in 2015 marked a watershed moment in acknowledging women's sexual health needs, even as it sparked ongoing conversations about the medicalization of desire.

Following flibanserin is bremelanotide, another groundbreaking drug introduced in 2019 as a treatment for HSDD. Unlike flibanserin, which is taken daily, bremelanotide is administered via subcutaneous injection on an as-needed basis. This flexibility allows women to use the medication in conjunction with their sexual activity, catering to the situational nature of sexual desire. Bremelanotide works by stimulating melanocortin receptors in the brain, which are associated with sexual arousal and desire. Its development was informed by studies that highlighted the role of these receptors in regulating sexual behavior, particularly in women.

The mechanism of action for bremelanotide differs significantly from that of flibanserin. By directly influencing the central nervous system's pathways related to arousal, bremelanotide provides a unique alternative for women who may not respond well to daily medication or who prefer a more situational approach. Initial clinical trials indicated that bremelanotide could significantly enhance sexual desire and arousal, offering a much-needed option for women who experience HSDD. However, like flibanserin, bremelanotide is not without its side effects, which can include nausea, flushing, and headache. Its introduction further enriched the conversation about women's sexual health, challenging societal norms and encouraging women to seek solutions that resonate with their experiences.

Another category of medications that often comes up in discussions about female sexual health involves testosterone therapy. While testosterone is traditionally associated with male sexuality, its role in women's health is increasingly recognized. Testosterone is produced in smaller quantities in women but plays a crucial role in libido, sexual function, and overall well-being. Some women experience a decline in testosterone levels due to aging, hormonal changes, or other medical conditions, which can lead to diminished sexual desire.

While testosterone therapy is not officially approved specifically for women, some healthcare providers prescribe it off-label for women experiencing low libido. Research suggests that testosterone can positively influence sexual desire and satisfaction in women, but its use remains controversial. The debate revolves around the risks and benefits, potential side effects (such as acne, hair growth, and mood changes), and the ethical implications of using hormone therapy in women. The lack of standardized guidelines further complicates the situation, making it imperative for women to consult knowledgeable healthcare professionals who can navigate these complex issues.

In addition to these primary medications, there are also emerging options that explore different mechanisms to enhance female sexual health. One such area of interest involves the use of herbal supplements and nutraceuticals. While not classified as traditional pharmaceuticals, these products have gained popularity among women seeking alternatives or complementary approaches to improving sexual desire. Some herbal supplements, such as ginseng, maca root, and tribulus terrestris, have been touted for their potential aphrodisiac properties. However, scientific evidence supporting their effectiveness is limited and often mixed, underscoring the importance of caution when considering these options.

Moreover, recent developments in clinical research have led to the exploration of other innovative treatments, such as vaginal rejuvenation therapies and platelet-rich plasma (PRP) treatments. Vaginal rejuvenation, which can involve surgical or non-surgical procedures, aims to enhance sexual function by addressing issues related to vaginal dryness, atrophy, or laxity. PRP treatments, often referred to as the "O-Shot," involve injecting platelet-rich plasma derived from the patient's blood into specific areas to promote tissue regeneration and improve sexual response. While these treatments are still relatively new and require more extensive research, they reflect the growing recognition of the need for diverse approaches to female sexual health.

As we consider the various types of Lady Era drugs and treatments, it is essential to recognize the broader context in which they exist. The societal narrative surrounding women's sexuality has historically been fraught with stigma and misunderstanding, often leading to a reluctance to address female sexual health openly. The introduction of these medications represents a significant shift, empowering women to seek solutions tailored to their needs. However, the ongoing conversation about their use must balance the potential benefits with considerations of safety, ethics, and individual experiences.

Moreover, the quest for effective treatments should not overshadow the importance of holistic approaches to sexual health. Education, communication, and emotional well-being are crucial components of a woman's sexual experience. Many women may find that therapy, relationship counseling, or support groups provide valuable insights and resources that medication alone cannot fulfill. By fostering a more comprehensive understanding of female sexuality, we can create an environment that encourages women to explore their desires, communicate openly with partners, and advocate for their health.

In conclusion, the landscape of Lady Era drugs encompasses a variety of medications and treatments, each reflecting the complexity of female sexuality and the ongoing journey to address women's health needs. Flibanserin and bremelanotide have set the stage for a more nuanced understanding of sexual desire, while the exploration of testosterone therapy, herbal supplements, and emerging treatments illustrates the diversity of options available. As research continues to evolve, it is vital to maintain an open dialogue about the implications of these drugs and to empower women to make informed decisions about their sexual health. In the following chapters, we will delve into the safety and side effects of these medications, the societal implications of their use, and personal narratives that illuminate the real-world experiences of women navigating this intricate landscape.

Chapter Four

Safety and Side Effects

When discussing Lady Era drugs, a crucial aspect to consider is their safety and potential side effects. These medications, designed to enhance female sexual health, have opened the door to a more nuanced conversation about women's needs and desires. However, as with any pharmacological intervention, it is imperative to understand both the benefits and the risks associated with these treatments.

The safety profiles of drugs like flibanserin and bremelanotide have been the subject of extensive clinical trials and ongoing research, aimed at assessing their long-term effects and potential complications. Flibanserin, the first drug approved specifically for hypoactive sexual desire disorder (HSDD), has been scrutinized for its side effects, which include dizziness, fatigue, nausea, and potential risks when combined with alcohol. In clinical studies, participants reported experiencing adverse reactions at rates significantly higher than those who received a placebo. For instance, dizziness and drowsiness can impair a woman's ability to perform daily tasks, raising concerns about safety, especially in situations that require alertness, such as driving or operating machinery.

Perhaps the most significant concern with flibanserin involves its interaction with alcohol. The FDA has mandated that women refrain from drinking alcohol while taking the medication due to the increased risk of severe hypotension and syncope (fainting). This caution reflects a broader challenge in the medical community regarding the balance between treating sexual dysfunction and ensuring patient safety. Many women may already experience social pressures surrounding their sexuality, and the prohibition of alcohol can complicate social interactions, further contributing to feelings of isolation or frustration.

Bremelanotide, introduced later as an on-demand treatment for HSDD, presents its own set of potential side effects. While it offers flexibility for women who prefer to take a medication only as needed, common side effects include nausea, flushing, headache, and injection site reactions. Clinical trials have indicated that nausea can be particularly bothersome, affecting the overall experience of using the medication. For some women, the discomfort associated with these side effects may outweigh the potential benefits of enhanced sexual desire, prompting a critical examination of the medication's overall utility.

It's also essential to consider the psychological dimensions of using these medications. The decision to pursue treatment for HSDD is often accompanied by emotional and relational factors. Women may already experience anxiety related to their sexual health, and the side effects of these drugs can exacerbate feelings of self-consciousness or inadequacy. For instance, a woman who experiences nausea or dizziness after taking flibanserin may become increasingly anxious about engaging in sexual activity, inadvertently perpetuating a cycle of dysfunction. This highlights the importance of addressing not only the physiological aspects of sexual health but also the emotional and psychological implications of treatment.

The safety profiles of these medications have prompted important discussions within the medical community regarding the need for comprehensive patient education. Women should be informed about the potential risks and side effects associated with any medication they consider. Open communication between healthcare providers and patients is vital in helping women make informed choices about their treatment options. This dialogue should include discussions about lifestyle factors that may influence the effectiveness and safety of these medications, such as alcohol consumption, dietary habits, and underlying health conditions.

In addition to the immediate side effects, long-term safety remains a significant area of concern. Research on the long-term effects of flibanserin and bremelanotide is still in its early stages. While short-term studies have provided valuable insights, the need for ongoing monitoring of patients using these medications is crucial. Longitudinal studies that track the experiences of women over extended periods will help clarify the potential for cumulative effects, including changes in mental health, relationship dynamics, and overall quality of life.

Beyond the specific medications, the broader context of women's health and safety is essential to consider. The historical neglect of female sexual health has led to a medical environment where many women's issues remain under-researched. This lack of attention to women's health can have real implications for the safety and efficacy of treatments. For instance, conditions such as hormonal imbalances, psychological factors like anxiety or depression, and the influence of life events (e.g., childbirth, menopause) can all affect a woman's sexual health and how she responds to medication. As research continues to evolve, it will be crucial to take a more holistic approach to women's sexual health, addressing these multifaceted factors.

Moreover, discussions around safety and side effects often intersect with broader societal implications. The medicalization of female desire raises important ethical questions about the pressures women may face to conform to societal expectations regarding sexual performance and satisfaction. The introduction of Lady Era drugs can inadvertently contribute to a narrative that positions sexual enhancement as a necessity rather than a choice, leading to increased scrutiny on women who may choose not to pursue pharmaceutical solutions. This dynamic underscores the importance of fostering a cultural environment where women feel empowered to discuss their needs openly, without the stigma or pressure to conform to prescribed ideals of femininity and sexual performance.

Additionally, there is a growing recognition of the need for more comprehensive studies that include diverse populations in clinical trials. Historically, medical research has often centered on homogeneous groups, leading to gaps in understanding how different demographics—such as age, race, and socioeconomic status—respond to treatments. A more inclusive approach to research will enhance the safety and efficacy of Lady Era drugs by ensuring that a broader range of experiences and health needs are addressed.

In conclusion, the safety and side effects of Lady Era drugs like flibanserin and bremelanotide reflect a complex interplay of biological, psychological, and social factors. While these medications offer new avenues for addressing female sexual health, their use comes with important considerations that must not be overlooked. Comprehensive patient education, ongoing research, and open dialogue within the medical community are vital to navigating the intricacies of women's health. As we move forward in this discussion, it is essential to acknowledge the broader societal implications of these medications, fostering an environment where women can make informed choices about their sexual health without pressure or stigma. In the following chapters, we will explore the societal implications of these drugs, personal narratives that illuminate the real-world experiences of women, and alternative approaches that empower women to take control of their sexual health journeys.

Chapter Five

Societal Implications

The introduction and ongoing use of Lady Era drugs, particularly those designed to address female sexual dysfunction, carry profound societal implications that extend far beyond individual health outcomes. As these medications reshape conversations about women's sexual health, they also challenge long-standing societal norms and perceptions regarding female desire, autonomy, and well-being. The impact of these drugs reverberates through cultural attitudes, healthcare practices, and discussions about gender equity, ultimately influencing how society views women's sexuality as a whole.

Historically, women's sexual health has often been marginalized, perceived through a lens of stigma and misunderstanding. For centuries, societal norms dictated that female sexuality should be restrained or hidden, with open discussions considered taboo. The emergence of Lady Era drugs represents a significant shift in this narrative, as they validate the existence of female sexual desire and the need for treatment options. This recognition is not merely a medical advancement; it signifies a cultural turning point where women can assert their rights to experience sexual pleasure and seek solutions to enhance their sexual well-being.

However, the introduction of these drugs is not without its controversies. The medicalization of female sexual desire raises critical questions about societal pressures and expectations surrounding women's sexuality. On one hand, medications like flibanserin and bremelanotide empower women to reclaim their sexual health. On the other hand, there is a concern that these drugs may inadvertently contribute to a narrative that positions sexual enhancement as a necessity rather than a personal choice. This creates a dichotomy where women may feel compelled to seek pharmaceutical solutions in order to conform to societal ideals of sexuality and performance. Such pressures can lead to feelings of inadequacy in those who do not feel the need for medication or who do not respond positively to these treatments.

The commercialization of female sexual health through the lens of Lady Era drugs has implications for how companies market these medications. Pharmaceutical advertising often targets women's insecurities, reinforcing the idea that sexual desire is a measure of a woman's worth or femininity. Advertisements might portray an idealized version of sexual relationships, implying that medications are a quick fix for deeper relational or emotional issues. This kind of marketing can exacerbate feelings of self-doubt and inadequacy among women, particularly those struggling with their sexual health or experiencing challenges in intimate relationships. The message can become one of comparison—encouraging women to measure their experiences against an often unrealistic standard, thereby fueling the cycle of dissatisfaction.

Furthermore, the discourse surrounding Lady Era drugs also intersects with broader discussions about gender equity in healthcare. Historically, medical research has predominantly focused on male sexual health, often sidelining the unique needs of women. The introduction of these medications represents an important step toward rectifying this imbalance, as it highlights the need for more research and understanding of female sexuality. However, while the availability of Lady Era drugs is a positive development, it does not absolve the medical community of its responsibility to address the underlying issues that contribute to sexual dysfunction.

The existence of these drugs prompts a deeper examination of healthcare accessibility and equity. Not all women have equal access to these medications, which can be influenced by factors such as socioeconomic status, geographic location, and healthcare coverage. Many women face barriers in accessing appropriate medical care, whether due to financial constraints, lack of knowledgeable healthcare providers, or cultural stigmas surrounding sexual health. As these medications become more widely available, it is crucial to advocate for equitable access so that all women can benefit from advancements in sexual health care.

The societal implications of Lady Era drugs also extend into the realm of education and communication about sexual health. The conversation surrounding these medications can serve as a catalyst for broader discussions about female sexuality, reproductive health, and the importance of open dialogue. Educating women and their partners about the complexities of sexual desire and the available treatment options can help foster a more supportive environment. Comprehensive sexual health education that includes discussions about emotional and relational factors can empower women to understand their bodies and advocate for their needs.

Moreover, the emergence of Lady Era drugs has the potential to influence the way healthcare providers approach discussions about female sexual health. As awareness of these medications grows, there is an opportunity for healthcare professionals to engage in more meaningful conversations with their patients. This includes recognizing the emotional and psychological components of sexual health, validating women's experiences, and offering holistic treatment options that go beyond pharmaceuticals.

The narrative surrounding female desire is also evolving in popular culture, thanks in part to the visibility created by the introduction of Lady Era drugs. As women increasingly speak out about their sexual health and experiences, there is a growing movement toward destigmatizing female desire. Public discourse—through social media, literature, and advocacy—plays a vital role in normalizing conversations about women's sexuality, encouraging openness, and challenging societal norms. This shift can empower future generations to approach their sexual health with confidence, reducing the stigma that has historically surrounded these discussions.

While the introduction of Lady Era drugs has brought about significant change, it is essential to recognize that these medications are not a panacea. They are one piece of a larger puzzle that includes emotional health, relationship dynamics, and cultural attitudes toward female sexuality. As society continues to grapple with the complexities of women's sexual health, ongoing conversations about the implications of these drugs will be vital.

In conclusion, the societal implications of Lady Era drugs extend far beyond the individual experiences of those who use them. They challenge long-standing norms surrounding female desire, raise important questions about healthcare access and equity, and foster opportunities for open dialogue about women's sexual health. As these medications reshape the narrative around female sexuality, it is crucial to approach the conversation with sensitivity and an understanding of the broader cultural context. The ongoing evolution of this discourse has the potential to empower women, promote equity in healthcare, and ultimately transform societal attitudes toward female desire and well-being. In the subsequent chapters, we will delve into personal narratives that illuminate the experiences of women navigating these complexities and explore alternative approaches to sexual health that prioritize empowerment and informed choice.

Chapter Six

Personal Experiences: Societal Implications

Personal narratives play a crucial role in understanding the societal implications of Lady Era drugs and how they intersect with women's lives. Individual experiences often illuminate the broader cultural and social dynamics that shape attitudes toward female sexuality, desire, and health. By sharing stories from diverse women who have navigated the landscape of sexual health, we can gain insight into the complexities of their journeys, the challenges they face, and the impact of these medications on their lives.

One woman's experience highlights the internal conflict that many face when considering treatment for hypoactive sexual desire disorder (HSDD). She recalls a long struggle with diminished libido, which she attributed to various life stressors, including work pressures, parenting responsibilities, and the emotional toll of her relationship. After much deliberation, she consulted her healthcare provider about flibanserin, the first drug approved for HSDD. While she was initially hopeful about the medication, she also grappled with societal messages that framed sexual desire as a marker of femininity.

The societal narrative surrounding women's sexuality often portrays desire as an innate trait, one that should be consistently present and easily accessible. This woman found herself questioning whether her struggles with sexual desire made her less of a woman. The societal expectation that women should always be sexually available or desirous contributed to her feelings of inadequacy. Ultimately, her decision to try flibanserin was rooted in a desire to reclaim her sexual identity, but it was fraught with anxiety about how others would perceive her choices.

Another woman's story brings to light the importance of open communication about sexual health. After experiencing a decline in sexual desire post-menopause, she felt isolated and unsure of how to approach the topic with her partner. The stigma surrounding female sexuality made her reluctant to discuss her needs, leading to misunderstandings and frustration in her relationship. When she learned about bremelanotide, she felt a sense of relief, viewing it as a potential solution to her difficulties.

However, her journey did not end with the medication. The decision to try bremelanotide prompted a candid conversation with her partner, allowing them to address not only her sexual health but also the emotional aspects of their intimacy. This dialogue was transformative, breaking down barriers that had been built over years of unspoken discomfort. Her experience illustrates how Lady Era drugs can serve as a catalyst for deeper connections and more honest conversations about sexual health, ultimately enriching relationships and challenging societal norms that discourage open discussion.

The narratives of women who have utilized these medications also reflect the need for better education and awareness around female sexual health. One woman shared her frustration with the lack of information available about HSDD and the available treatment options. Despite her struggles, she felt ill-equipped to navigate the healthcare system, largely due to the stigma surrounding discussions of female desire. Her experience highlights a critical gap in sexual health education that affects many women.

This gap often leaves women feeling unsupported and uninformed, reinforcing societal messages that their desires are unworthy of attention or discussion. When she finally learned about flibanserin, she realized the importance of advocating for herself and seeking knowledge about her body. This shift empowered her not only to explore treatment options but also to share her story with other women, helping to foster a sense of community and collective understanding around sexual health issues.

The societal implications of Lady Era drugs are further compounded by the intersection of race, culture, and socioeconomic status. One woman of color recounted her experience navigating healthcare as a member of a marginalized community. She expressed how cultural taboos around sexuality often prevented open discussions with healthcare providers, leaving her feeling unheard and misunderstood. The stigma surrounding both her race and her sexuality created barriers that influenced her ability to seek help for her sexual dysfunction.

When she finally learned about bremelanotide, she felt a mixture of hope and skepticism. The historical neglect of women's health issues in her community led her to question whether these drugs would truly address her needs or simply perpetuate existing inequalities. Her story underscores the importance of culturally competent care and the necessity for healthcare providers to approach discussions about female sexual health with sensitivity to the unique challenges faced by women from diverse backgrounds.

As these personal narratives reveal, the societal implications of Lady Era drugs extend far beyond the individual. They reflect the collective struggles women face in a world that often stigmatizes and marginalizes their experiences. The conversations sparked by these medications challenge societal norms, encourage openness, and promote a culture of acceptance around female desire and sexual health.

Moreover, the stories shared by these women highlight the importance of community and support networks in navigating sexual health challenges. Many women found solace and strength in connecting with others who shared similar experiences. Support groups, online forums, and social media platforms have become valuable resources, allowing women to exchange information, share their journeys, and foster a sense of belonging. This sense of community is crucial in dismantling the stigma surrounding female sexuality and empowering women to advocate for their health.

In conclusion, personal experiences related to Lady Era drugs provide valuable insights into the societal implications of these medications. The stories of women navigating sexual health challenges reflect broader cultural attitudes toward female desire, the importance of open communication, and the necessity of equitable access to care. As these narratives unfold, they underscore the urgent need for a cultural shift that embraces female sexuality, encourages honest discussions, and empowers women to seek the care they deserve. The journey toward understanding and addressing women's sexual health is ongoing, and the experiences shared by these women will continue to shape the conversation, fostering a more inclusive and supportive environment for all. In the following chapters, we will explore alternative approaches to sexual health that prioritize empowerment and informed choice, alongside further discussions on the importance of comprehensive sexual health education.

www.ingramcontent.com/pod-product-compliance
Lightning Source LLC
Chambersburg PA
CBHW081020240526
45471CB00018B/3920